Colour **Aids**

Clinical Signs

Peter C. Hayes BMSc MD MRCP

Lecturer in Medicine,
Department of Medicine,
Royal Infirmary,
Edinburgh, UK

Derek Bell BSc MD MRCP

Senior Registrar,
Department of Thoracic Medicine,
Central Middlesex Hospital,
London, UK

Churchill Livingstone

EDINBURGH LONDON MELBOURNE AND NEW YORK 1990

Preface

The intention of this book is to illustrate many of the commoner classical signs. This, we believe, is useful both for the undergraduate, and for the doctor revising for such examinations as the MRCP. It is our aim to illustrate typical examples of clinical signs rather than the gross extremes. This book would not have been possible without help from many of our colleagues in providing photographs. We would like to thank Dr Gordon Scott, Dr Andrew Williams, Dr Wilfred Treasure, Dr Christopher Thompson, Dr Andrew Collier, Dr Kelvin Palmer, Mr Stephen Nixon, Dr Margaret MacIntyre, Dr Michael Hayes, the Dermatology Department, Ninewells Hospital, Dundee, the Gastrointestinal Unit, Western General Hospital, Edinburgh and the Department of Respiratory Medicine, Central Middlesex Hospital, London.

Edinburgh and London, 1990   P.C.H.
D.B.

Contents

General Signs (1)

Finger clubbing

This is an important clinical sign since its presence commonly indicates serious underlying disease. It should be specifically looked for and its presence or absence recorded.

Definition

The earliest change in the development of finger clubbing is swelling of the soft tissue at the base of the nail, with increased nail bed fluctuation (Fig. 1). As this progresses, loss of the nail bed angle occurs (Fig. 2) and, later, increased curvature of the long axis of the nail. Finally, swelling of the finger pulp in all dimensions occurs (Fig. 3), with or without the development of hypertrophic pulmonary osteoarthropathy. This latter condition is recognised clinically as tender wrists, and radiologically by periosteal elevation.

Causes

Diseases associated with clubbing can be divided into four main groups:
1. Respiratory, e.g. bronchial carcinoma, bronchiectasis and fibrosing alveolitis.
2. Gastrointestinal, e.g. malabsorption, Crohn's disease and cirrhosis.
3. Cardiac, e.g. cyanotic congenital heart disease and infective endocarditis.
4. Miscellaneous, e.g. thyrotoxicosis, branchial arteriovenous fistula (one hand only) and familial.

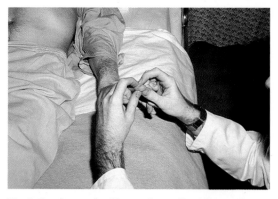

Fig. 1 Correct method for testing nailbed fluctuation.

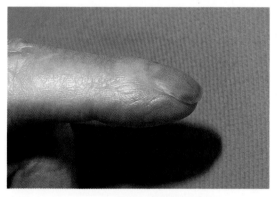

Fig. 2 Loss of nail bed angle in finger clubbing.

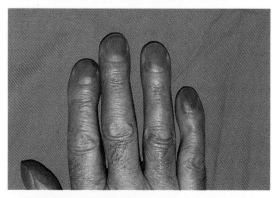

Fig. 3 Swelling of the finger pulp in all directions in final stages of finger clubbing.

General Signs (2)

Nails

Examination of the nails can often provide information as to underlying disease.

Clinical signs and associated disorders

Pseudo-clubbing
Finger clubbing is described on p. 1, but a clubbing of similar appearance is seen in hyperparathyroidism due to resorption of the terminal phalanges (Fig. 4).

Leukonychia
This is a white discolouration of the nails which occurs in hypoalbuminaemia such as is common in liver disease (Fig. 90).

Splinter haemorrhages
Longitudinal splinter haemorrhages occur in endocarditis and with trauma. Transverse haemorrhages occur in trichinosis.

Onycholysis
Lifting of the nail from its bed occurs in hyperthyroidism, psoriasis (Fig. 5), eczema and fungal infections. The latter is commoner in hypoparathyroidism (Fig. 6).

Koilonychia
Spoon-shaped nails were once recognised as being associated with iron-deficiency anaemia, but a direct relationship is no longer accepted.

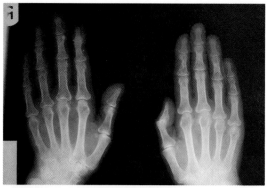

Fig. 4 Resorption of terminal phalanges due to hyperparathyroidism.

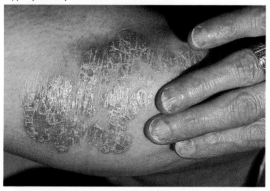

Fig. 5 Onycholysis as occurs in psoriasis.

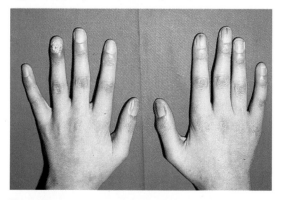

Fig. 6 Onycholysis due to hypoparathyroidism.

General Signs (3)

Nails (contd)

Pitting
This occurs in psoriasis (Fig. 7) and may be associated with arthropathy of the affected fingers.

Nail bed infarcts
These occur in vasculitides, such as systemic lupus erythematosus (SLE), rheumatoid disease and polyarteritis nodosa.

Dystrophia
This may occur as a result of trauma or in syndromes such as Cronkite-Canada syndrome, which occurs along with alopecia, pigmentation and intestinal polyps (Fig. 8). Eczema may also be associated with nail dystrophy.

Beau's lines
These are transverse depressions resulting from temporary disturbance in nail growth, as occurs with acute illness.

Nail-patella syndrome
In this disorder, split and deformed nails are associated with rudimentary patellas, iliac horns and mild, but sometimes progressive, glomerulonephritis.

Smooth nails
These are associated with pruritus, where the nails are smoothed by chronic scratching.

Nail edge abnormalities
Abnormalities of the lateral nail fold are common and include such disorders as ingrowing toenail and paronychia. Less common signs, such as periungual fibromas, may accompany underlying disorders such as tuberous sclerosis (Fig. 9). The nail edges are also common sites for viral warts (p. 9).

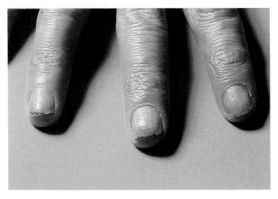

Fig. 7 Pitting of nails in psoriasis.

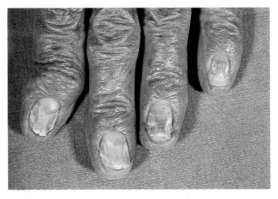

Fig. 8 Nail dystrophy in Cronkite-Canada syndrome.

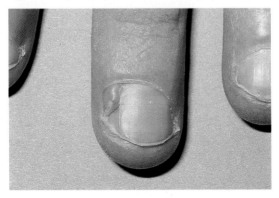

Fig. 9 Periungal fibroma accompanying tuberous sclerosis.

| # General Signs (4)

Hands and feet

The hands and feet should be examined in all patients, irrespective of their complaint, as clues to the underlying disorder are often found.

Palmar erythema
This is a patchy, bright-red disclouration of the hypothenar eminence of the palms which occurs most often in alcoholic cirrhosis, rheumatoid arthritis, thyrotoxicosis and pregnancy.

Dupuytren's contracture
This is characterised by fibrosis of the palmar fascia, usually of the 4th or 5th fingers (Fig. 10), and is probably more common in alcoholic liver disease, although its prevalence in the healthy population is high.

Abnormal skin creases
The skin creases should be examined, as their colour may be useful in assessing the severity of anaemia. Abnormal patterns of folds such as the Simian crease, which is a feature of Down's syndrome, may be apparent.

Tremor
In thyrotoxicosis, a fine tremor may be evident and the hands are often warm and sweaty. A coarser tremor is seen in Parkinsonism, and a flapping tremor in liver failure and hypercapnia.

Palm abnormalities
The palms should also be inspected for such abnormalities as pompholyx (Fig. 11), a form of dermatitis which, although of unknown cause, may be associated with fungal infection of the feet.

Keratoderma blenorrhagica
This is a hyperkeratotic rash on the soles of the feet (Fig. 12), very similar to pustular psoriasis, and is characteristic of Reiter's syndrome.

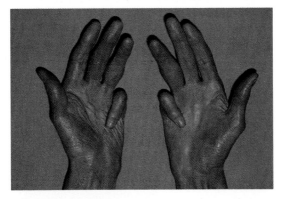

Fig. 10 Dupuytren's contracture.

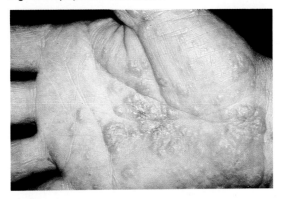

Fig. 11 Pompholyx affecting the palms.

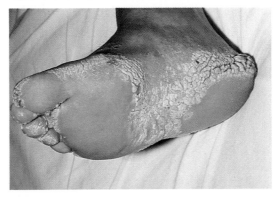

Fig. 12 Keratoderma blenorrhagica, characteristic of Reiter's syndrome.

General Signs (5)

Fingers

Deformities
Deformity should be looked for, and associated
tendon damage and joint subluxation (as occurs
in rheumatoid arthritis, p. 91) identified.
Deformity may also be due to such disorders as
scleroderma (Fig. 13), injury and burns. The webs
of the fingers and toes should be inspected for
fungal infection and scabies (Fig. 14).

Other abnormalities
Inspection may reveal other obvious
abnormalities, such as nicotine staining which
may be of relevance in patients being
investigated for pulmonary or vascular disease
(although the staining is often related more to the
manner of cigarette smoking than the intensity).

Muscle wasting
This occurs in rheumatoid arthritis, peripheral
nerve lesions (p. 89) and in old age. The pattern of
wasting provides evidence as to the cause, as
does any associated fasciculation.

Lumps
Heberden's nodes are palpable osteophytes on
the dorsal aspect of the base of the terminal
phalanx; they occur in patients with primary
osteoarthrosis. In this disorder, the hand may
have a 'square' appearance due to deformity of
the first carpometacarpal joint. Osler's nodes are
now rare, but are occasionally found in infective
endocarditis as tender lumps in the finger pulps.
Other lesions such as simple warts (Fig. 15) and
gouty tophi should be identified.

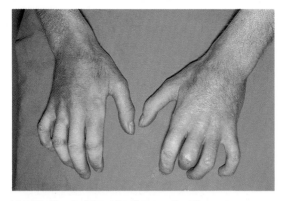

Fig. 13 Finger deformity due to scleroderma.

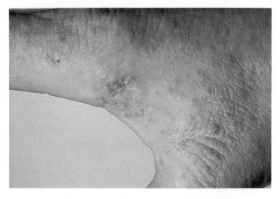

Fig. 14 Typical position of burrows in scabies.

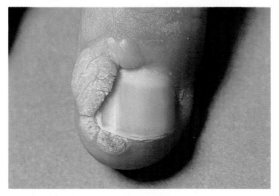

Fig. 15 Simple wart.

General Signs (6)

Skin

Skin lesions may represent cutaneous or systemic disease. Accurate description of the lesion is important and should include the type (e.g. macule, papule or petechiae), shape and distribution.

Primary skin disorders

Psoriasis
This affects 1–2% of the population. The lesions are often symmetrical and usually affect the scalp and extensor surfaces, but any area can be involved (Fig. 16). The lesions are erythematous and scaly, and psoriatic arthropathy occurs in 5% of patients, often associated with nail pitting. Other nail changes include oncholysis and thickening of the nail plate.

The cause of psoriasis is unknown and usually starts in adolescence.

Dermatitis and eczema
The terms are often used synonymously to indicate the common pattern of skin change in response to irritation. Atopic eczema (Fig. 17) affects 1–3% of the population and often starts in childhood. A family history and associated hayfever or asthma is common.

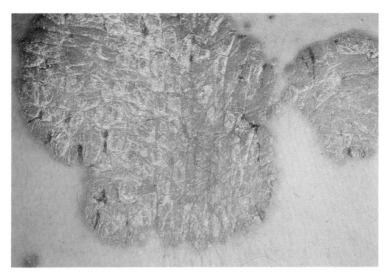

Fig. 16 Psoriasis plaque.

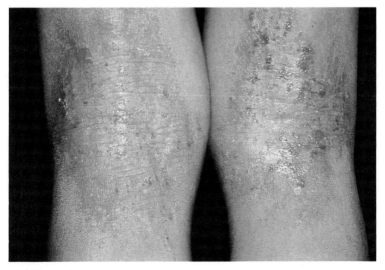

Fig. 17 Atopic eczema.

Skin (contd)

Drug eruptions
Drug hypersensitivity rashes are common and can be caused by almost any drug. The rashes may be erythematous, maculopapular, urticarial, bullous or purpuric. The most characteristic drug rash, erythema multiforme, (Fig. 18) may also be caused by herpes simplex or mycoplasma infection.

Others
There are numerous other common skin disorders; the most important include:
1. *Acne vulgaris:* particularly common in adolescent males, affecting the face, neck and shoulders. The cause is not absolutely understood, but is probably related to changes in sex hormones. In later life, acne vulgaris may be associated with Cushing's syndrome, diabetes and acromegaly.
2. *Pityriasis rosea:* a maculopapular rash over the trunk (Fig. 19), thighs and arms which is often preceeded by a 'herald patch' and rosacea affecting the nose, cheeks, chin and forehead.
   Less common disorders include lichen planus (Fig. 20), an inflammatory disorder of the epidermis of unknown cause, and congenital ichthyosis (Fig. 21).

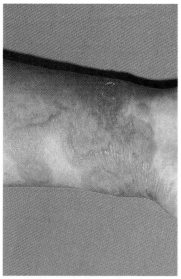

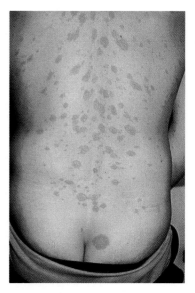

Fig. 18 Target lesions of erythema multiforme. Can be a sign of Stevens-Johnson syndrome if found in association with mouth ulcers.

Fig. 19 Pityriasis rosea.

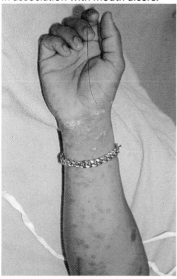

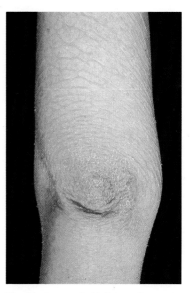

Fig. 20 Lichen planus. Note: papules can be mauve or violaceous.

Fig. 21 Congenital ichthyosis.

Skin (contd)

Connective tissue disease
The skin is often involved in connective tissue disorders, particularly systemic lupus erythematosus, dermatomyositis and scleroderma.

Vascular disorders
Vascular lesions are common. Bleeding into the skin may occur as petechiae (1–3 mm), purpura or ecchymoses. These may reflect thrombocytopenia, coagulopathy or blood vessel abnormality as occurs in scurvy (Fig. 22), and vasculitides such as Henoch-Schonlein purpura (Fig. 23). This latter condition is a generalised vasculitis which results in glomerulonephritis, arthralgia, and abdominal pain, as well as purpura. It is commonest in children, and the treatment is symptomatic in the majority.

Urticaria may occur as a result of local insult, or increased vascular reactivity (Fig. 24) which can produce the phenomenon of dermatographia (Fig. 25, p. 18).

Another skin manifestation of vascular disease is livedo reticularis, which should be distinguished from the more common erythema abigne.

A further common skin disorder associated with vascular disease is eczema over the shin, frequently seen in patients with chronic venous insufficiency. Ulcers in this disorder are common and notoriously slow to heal.

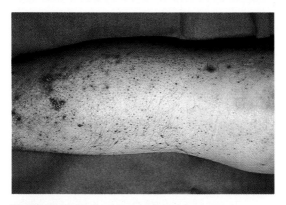

Fig. 22 Perifollicular haemorrhages in scurvy.

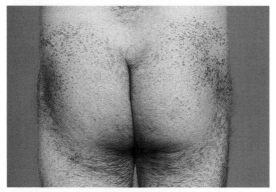

Fig. 23 Typical distribution of purpuric rash in Henoch-Schonlein purpura.

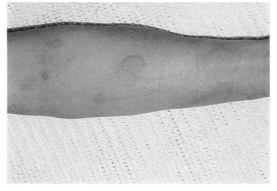
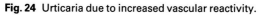

Fig. 24 Urticaria due to increased vascular reactivity.

Skin (contd)

Infection
The skin is commonly involved with infectious processes either directly or indirectly. Primary skin infections can largely be broken down into bacterial and viral.

1. *Bacterial.* Staphylococcal and streptococcal organisms are amongst the commonest bacteria involved, the second classically producing cellulitis and erysipelas (Fig. 26). This latter most often affects the legs or face.
2. *Viral.* The most common viral infections of the skin in adults are herpes simplex (Fig. 78, p. 54) and herpes zoster (Fig. 27). The latter most often affects the dermatomes over the chest and abdomen, and, because it is frequently painful, should be remembered as a cause of chest and abdominal pain (particularly in the phase before the tell-tale rash appears).

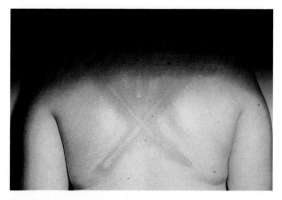

Fig. 25 Dermatographia in urticaria.

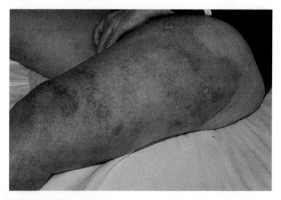

Fig. 26 Erysipelas.

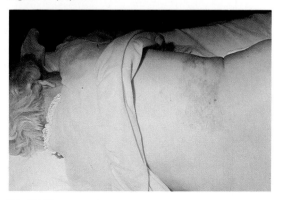

Fig. 27 Herpes zoster.

General Signs (10)

Skin pigmentation

Normal skin colour is dependent upon three factors: melanin, haemoglobin (oxidised and reduced) and carotene. Changes in colour are due to alterations in the normal ratio of these components.

Increased pigmentation
Yellow discolouration occurs due to bilirubin in hepatobiliary disease or haemolysis, or due to carotene from excessive consumption of carotenoid foods, myxoedema or renal failure. Increased pigmentation due to haemoglobin occurs in polycythaemia, cyanosis and met-, sulph- and carboxy-haemoglobinaemia. Increased melanin pigmentation occurs in sun tanning, haemochromatosis and Addison's disease (Fig. 28), and ectopic ACTH syndrome (Fig. 29). Increased pigmentation may be localised in naevi, heavy-metal poisoning, melanomas and haemangiomas, and acanthosis nigricans (p. 27).

Decreased pigmentation
The commonest cause is anaemia. Others include circulatory insufficiency and oedema. Localised decreased pigmentation occurs in scar tissue and vitiligo (Fig. 30).

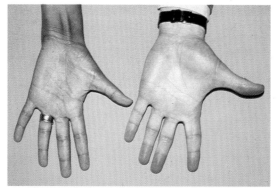

Fig. 28 Increased melanin pigmentation in Addison's Disease. Normal hand for comparison on the right.

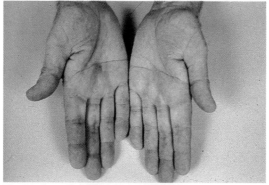

Fig. 29 Ectopic ACTH syndrome evidenced by increased melanin pigmentation.

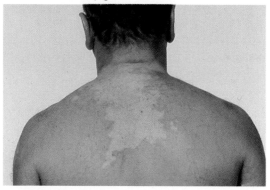

Fig. 30 Vitilgo with a localised decrease in skin pigmentation.

Bullous diseases

Bullous skin disorders are relatively uncommon. They include the following:

Dermatitis herpetiformis
This is an intensely itchy skin eruption which appears to be related to gluten enteropathy. The rash (Fig. 31) occurs typically on the elbows, shoulders, knees and sacral areas. The bowel lesion closely resembles coeliac disease with villous atrophy, and both the bowel and the skin eruption settle with strict adherence to a glute-free diet.

Pemphigus vulgaris and pemphigoid
A further, uncommon, bullous skin disorder is pemphigus vulgaris (Fig. 32), which occurs in middle age and features superficial blisters affecting the epidermis. Pemphigoid (Fig. 33) occurs in the elderly and affects the deeper layer between the dermis and epidermis. In both pemphigoid and pemphigus, a typical deposition of immunoglobulin can be demonstrated histologically, and steroid therapy is effective (although large doses may be required in pemphigus).

The most gross form of bullous disorder is toxic epidermal necrolysis, which in adults is usually the result of staphylococcal infection (Fig. 34).

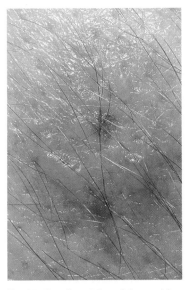

Fig. 31 Small vesicles of dermatitis herpetiformis.

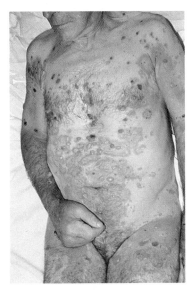

Fig. 32 Superficial blisters of pemphigus vulgaris.

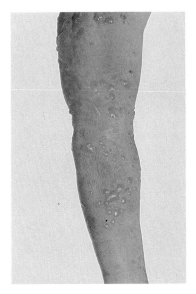

Fig. 33 Pemphigoid.

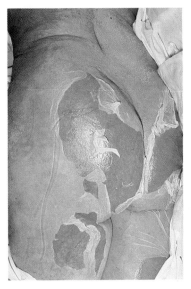

Fig. 34 Toxic epidermal necrolysis.

Skin lumps

General

Inspection of the skin commonly reveals clues of underlying systemic disease. Localised skin lumps should be characterised by site, position (e.g. skin, subcutaneous tissue, muscle or bone), shape, size, consistency and tenderness. They can broadly be classed into benign, premalignant and malignant lesions.

Benign

These may be:
1. Congenital, such as strawberry naevi (Fig. 35) which grow rapidly in babies but usually resolve before adolescence.
2. Genetically determined, such as the soft pedunculated benign tumours in von Recklinghausen's disease (Fig. 36).
3. Aquired, such as seborrhoeic keratoses (Fig. 37), one of the commonest benign tumours in the elderly.

Some benign tumours, such as keratoacanthoma, closely resemble malignant lesions (Fig. 38). These usually develop in light-exposed areas, grow rapidly and, if left untreated, will resolve spontaneously.

Other benign lesions include granuloma annulare (p. 99), which start as nodules and spread out to develop crater-shaped lumps. Pyogenic granulomas (Fig. 39, p. 26) are rapid proliferations of granulation tissue which may follow minor injury.

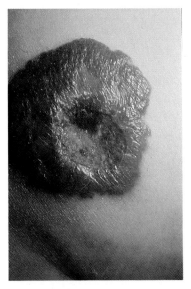

Fig. 35 Strawberry naevus.

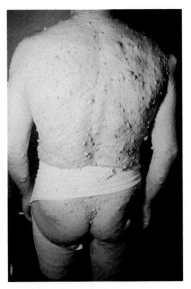

Fig. 36 Benign tumours of von Recklinghausen's disease.

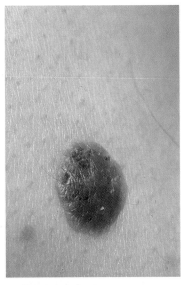

Fig. 37 Seborrhoeic keratosis.

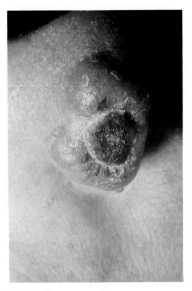

Fig. 38 Keratoacanthoma.

Skin lumps (contd)

Premalignant

These include Bowen's disease (p. 27), leukoplakia (p. 33) and solar keratoses.

Malignant

The most sinister skin malignancy is the melanoma (Fig. 40). It is believed that about half of these develop from existing moles, and suspicious lesions which grow in size, ulcerate or bleed should be removed early.

Squamous-cell carcinoma
This variety (Fig. 41) develops in skin damaged by ultra-violet light, radiation or trauma. Those on the ears, lips and genitals metastasize early in comparison to those which develop in sunlight-damaged regions.

Basal-cell carcinoma
Also known as rodent ulcer, this is a slow-growing, locally destructive tumour which rarely metastasizes. It is the commonest skin tumour and arises from the basal layer of the epidermis. It is most frequently found on the face, but may also arise from scars or areas of radiation damage to the skin. Curettage may be curative for small tumours, whilst larger lesions require wider excision or radiotherapy.

Mycosis fungoides
This is a slowly growing reticulosis, which presents with telangiectatic scaly patches, initially, before enlarging and becoming infiltrative (Fig. 42).

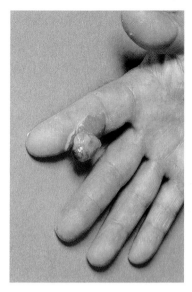

Fig. 39 Pyogenic granulomas.

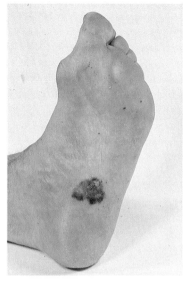

Fig. 40 Malignant melanoma.

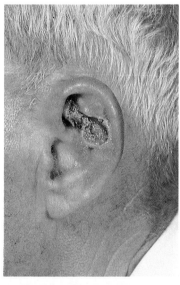

Fig. 41 Squamous-cell carcinoma.

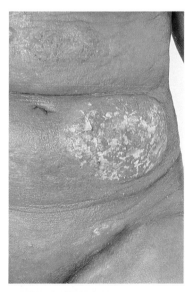

Fig. 42 Large area of mycosis fungoides on abdomen. Usually well circumscribed and scaly.

Skin disorders associated with malignancy

Internal malignancy may present with cutaneous manifestations. The best known of these include:

Acanthosis nigricans
This may precede overt malignancy by years. It is characterised by thickening and darkening of the skin in the flexures, where the skin is often covered by brown papules or warts (Fig. 43). Minor forms may occur in adolescents, but when associated with malignancy the disorder is often marked and frequently affects the mucus membranes. It may also regress if the underlying tumour is treated successfully.

Aquired ichthyosis
This may also be a manifestation of underling malignancy, most often Hodgkin's disease. Dermatomyositis (Fig. 44) may also occur in patients with cancer, and again may precede the diagnosis of the underlying tumour by years and regress after treatment.

Bowen's disease
When not affecting skin damage by sunlight, this condition is strongly associated with internal malignancy (Fig. 45).

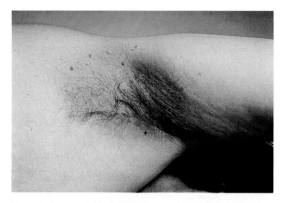

Fig. 43 Acanthosis nigricans.

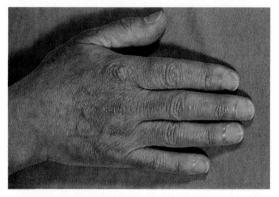

Fig. 44 Dermatomyositis.

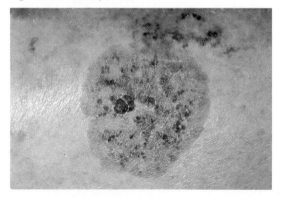

Fig. 45 Bowen's disease.

Eyes

Eyelids
Abnormalities include xanthelasma (p. 61),
swelling in myxoedema, allergy and local
infection, lid retraction in thyrotoxicosis, ptosis in
III nerve or cervical sympathetic chain lesions,
ectropion and entropion.

Sclera
Blue sclera are characteristic of osteogenesis
imperfecta (Fig. 46).

Cornea
A corneal arcus is common in the elderly and has
little significance. Calcification and Kayser-
Fleisher rings are seen on rare occasions.

Pupils
Pupil abnormalities are bilateral in pontine
haemorrhage or drug toxicity, and unilateral in III
cranial nerve or sympathetic chain lesions.

Lens
Cataracts occur in the elderly, diabetics, after
trauma and, rarely, with steroid therapy.

Fundi
Retinoscopy may reveal diabetes (p. 97),
hypertension or anaemia (Fig. 47). Papilloedema
(Fig. 48) should be looked for, as should less
common disorders such as retinitis pigmentosa.

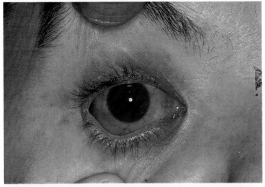

Fig. 46 Blue sclera, typically found in osteogenesis imperfecta.

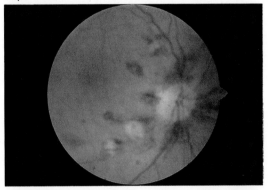

Fig. 47 Macular appearance of severe megaloblastic anaemia.

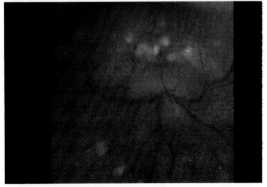

Fig. 48 Papilloedema

| # General Signs (16)

Mouth

The lips and mouth are the only readily visualised parts of the gastrointestinal tract and may provide clues to diseases in this system and elsewhere.

Lips
The lips should be inspected for such abnormalities as patches of pigmentation, as seen in Peutz-Jegher's syndrome (Fig. 49), an inherited disorder with multiple hamartomatous polyps throughout the GI tract which may present with bleeding and which have increased malignant potential. Vascular abnormalities, as occurs in hereditary haemorrhagic telangiectasia (Fig. 50), may be identified around the lips. Herpes simplex infections, or cold sores, commonly reappear in ill patients, especially those with pneumonia or who are immuno-suppressed.

Gums
The gums are also a common site of disease, the most common being gingivitis. Bleeding from the spongy gums of subjects with scurvy is now rare, as is the linear discolouration of lead poisoning. Hypertrophy of the gums may occur in some patients receiving phenytoin, and in acute leukaemia.

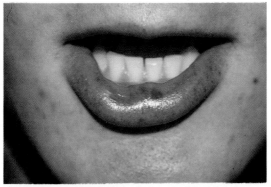

Fig. 49 Abnormal patches of pigmentation seen in Peutz-Jegher's syndrome.

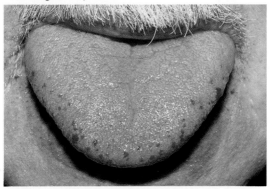

Fig. 50 Vascular abnormalities as seen in hereditary haemorrhagic telangiectasia.

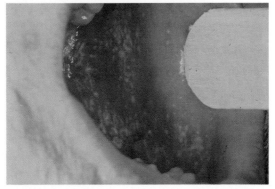

Fig. 51 Lichen planus.

Mouth (contd)

Buccal mucosa
The buccal mucosa is one of the best sites to look for cyanosis and, if present at this site, indicates central cyanosis. Lichen planus (Fig. 51, p. 32) may occur in the mouth, as may leukoplakia which is premalignant (Fig. 52). The presence of oral candidiasis should raise the question of AIDS. Although its presence alone does not indicate AIDS, it should stimulate the observer to investigate the oesophagus, as candidal oesophagitis correlates strongly with AIDS.

Tongue
The tongue should be inspected closely looking for glossitis (Fig. 53) as may occur in Vitamin B deficiency.

Teeth
Staining from smoking may be obvious, as may pitting and staining in fluorosis. Enamel hypoplasia occurs in association with tuberous sclerosis (Fig. 54). Infants of mothers treated with tetracycline during pregnancy may develop brown discolouration of their teeth.

Abnormalities around the mouth, such as perioral dermatitis, may be obvious. This condition is commonest in adolescent females and may complicate topical steroid use. Angular stomatitis is also common, particularly in the elderly, due to candidal infection.

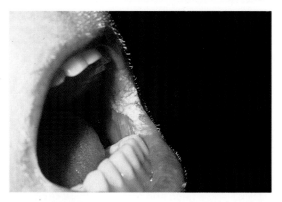

Fig. 52 Leukoplakia.

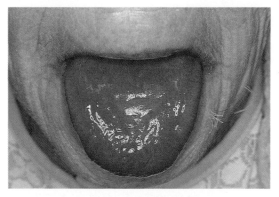

Fig. 53 Glossitis due to Vitamin B deficiency.

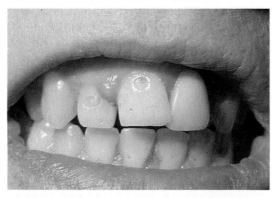

Fig. 54 Enamel hypoplasia in tuberous sclerosis.

Breasts

Breast disease is common, and breast cancer is the most frequent cancer in females (Fig. 55). It is an essential part of clinical examination that the breasts are closely inspected and palpated.

Head and neck

Inspection

The head and neck should be closely observed in all patients, and abnormalities such as tumours, raised JVP (Fig. 56), alopecia and syndromatic changes, such as myxoedema or acromegaly (Fig. 57), noted.

JVP

This should be examined with the patient at 45° and the biphasic slow pulsation looked for. The external jugular vein should not be used to assess pressure, as it can be influenced by extraneous factors. The vertical height should be measured from the sternal angle, and confirmation that the pulse is venous can be made by light compression at its base when filling is observed from above.

Palpation

The thyroid should be palpated from behind, and gland movement confirmed by the patient swallowing. Systematic examination of the lymph nodes is essential, whilst such abnormalities as surgical emphysema should be sought in appropriate cases.

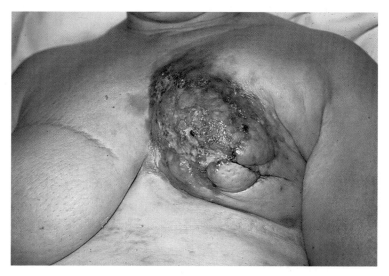

Fig. 55 Large fungating breast carcinoma.

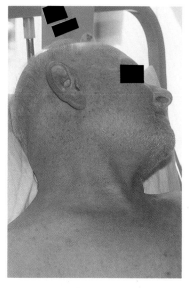

Fig. 56 Distension of internal jugular vein visible between the heads of the sterno-mastoid.

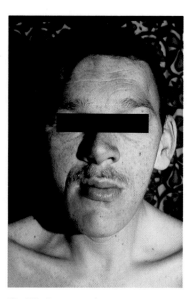

Fig. 57 Acromegaly.

Cardiovascular Disease (1)

Ischaemic heart disease

Incidence

This varies with population, being high in countries such as Scotland and Finland. It remains the commonest cause of death in Western society and is directly related to the prevalence of cigarette smoking.

Pathogenesis

The underlying mechanism is atheroma in the coronary arteries, and symptoms only develop when oxygen demand exceeds supply.

Clinical features

The diagnosis of ischaemic heart disease is based on the clinical history; often there is exertional angina or myocardial infarction. The description of crushing, central chest pain, often accompanied by a clenched fist held over the chest is characteristic (Fig. 58). Signs of associated diseases such as hypertension, hyperlipidaemia (Fig. 59), diabetes mellitus (p. 97) or cardiac failure may co-exist.

Risk factors

1. Smoking.
2. Hypertension.
3. Hypercholesterolaemia.
4. Obesity.
5. Diabetes mellitus.
6. Age.
7. Male sex.

Investigations

Abnormalities on a resting ECG may be diagnostic, but commonly these become obvious only with exercise. Coronary angiography is required in selected cases.

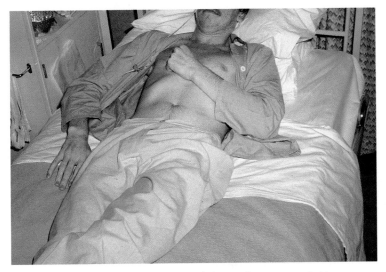

Fig. 58 A description of crushing, central chest pain accompanied by a clenched fist is characteristic of ischaemic heart disease.

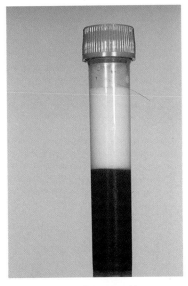

Fig. 59 Blood left to stand in severe hyperlipidaemia.

Valvular heart disease

Incidence

Mitral stenosis, the commonest cause only a few decades ago, has now been overtaken by aortic valve disease.

Aortic stenosis

In adults, the commonest cause is a calcified bicuspid valve.
Symptoms: angina pectoris, exertional dyspnoea and syncope.
Signs: a plateau pulse, thrusting apex beat, fourth heart sound and a characteristic harsh mid-systolic murmur.

Aortic regurgitation

Pure aortic regurgitation is seen in infective endocarditis, rheumatic fever, Marfan's syndrome, syphilis and ankylosing spondylitis.
Symptoms: usually asymptomatic until left ventricular failure develops.
Signs: collapsing pulse (Fig. 60), displaced apex beat and early diastolic murmur at the left lower sternal edge.

Mitral stenosis

This is usually rheumatic in origin.
Symptoms: exertional dyspnoea, haemoptysis, peripheral emboli and pulmonary hypertension.
Signs: atrial fibrillation, loud first heart sound, rumbling mid-diastolic murmur and a mitral facies (Fig. 61)

Mitral regurgitation

Causes include left ventricular dilatation, papillary muscle dysfunction, infective endocarditis and mitral valve prolapse.
Symptoms: Those of left ventricular failure (LVF).
Signs: pansystolic apical murmur radiating to the axilla.

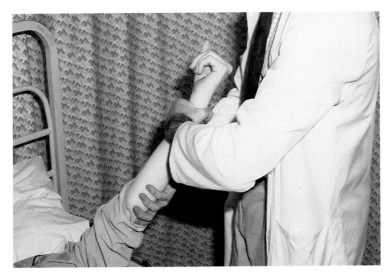

Fig. 60 The correct technique for assessing collapsing pulse.

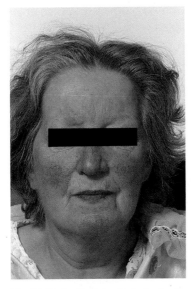

Fig. 61 Malar flush typical of mitral stenosis.

Cardiovascular Disease (3)

Infective endocarditis

Incidence

Approximately 6 cases/100 000 population per year in developed countries.

Pathogenesis

Is dependent on bacteraemia with colonisation of abnormal valves. *Streptococcus viridans* is the most common organism, with *Strept. faecalis* and Gram-negative organisms found more often in the elderly, and *Staph. pyogenes* post-operatively and in drug addicts.

Clinical features

Symptoms: general malaise, weight loss, sweats, myalgia and arthralgia, or with cardiac failure or systemic embolism.
Signs: finger clubbing, splinter haemorrhages (Fig. 62), vasculitic skin rash (Fig. 63), Roth spots or Osler's nodes (Fig. 64), haematuria and cardiac failure.

Investigations

Blood cultures on at least three occasions (whilst the patient is not on antibiotic therapy), full blood count and erythrocyte sedimentation rate (ESR), and urine microscopy for cellular casts. Echocardiography may demonstrate the valvular abnormality, but will identify vegetations in less than 30% of cases, and if negative does not exclude the diagnosis.

Treatment

At least four weeks of intravenous therapy with an antibiotic of proven efficacy against the organism responsible.

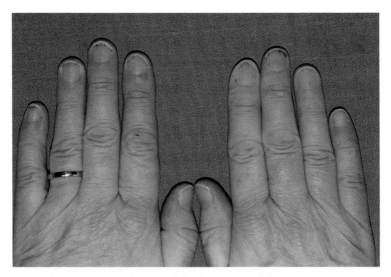

Fig. 62 Splinter haemorrhages in infective endocarditis.

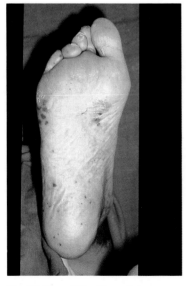

Fig. 63 Vasculitic skin rash in infective endocarditis.

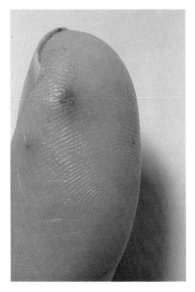

Fig. 64 Osler's nodes.

2 | Cardiovascular Disease (4)

Vascular disease

Arterial disease

The commonest disease of large- and medium-sized arteries is atheroma. Risk factors include smoking, hypertension, diabetes and hyperlipidaemia. Vessels commonly involved include the coronary, cerebral and lower limb arteries. The last produces the most obvious clinical signs—dry, peeling skin, ulceration (Fig. 65) and gangrene. Sudden occlusion of large arteries of the legs produces a cold, painful, pulseless limb.

Inflammatory arterial disease is less common and includes polyarteritis nodosa, giant cell arteritis and syphilis. Raynaud's syndrome, produced by spasm of small arteries due either to cold or emotional stimulus (Fig. 66), may give rise to trophic changes due to ischaemia.

Small vessel disease

This is most often due to diabetes mellitus or hypervicosity states, such as polycythaemia. The vasculitides may cause small focal areas of infarction, especially peripherally (Fig. 67). Less obvious lesions, involving internal organs such as the kidneys, may be inferred from the presence of haematuria. Involvement of the GI tract or liver may be apparent, with rectal bleeding or LFT abnormalities.

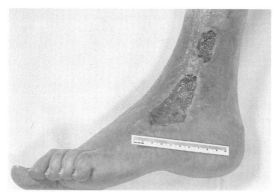

Fig. 65 Ulceration due to atheroma of lower limb, large- and medium-sized arteries.

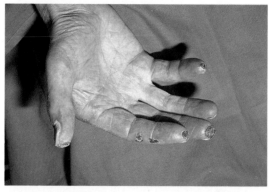

Fig. 66 Raynaud's syndrome with ischaemic ulcers.

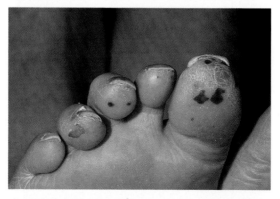

Fig. 67 Peripheral infarcts due to small vessel disease.

Vascular disease (contd)

Venous disease

Venous thrombosis in the lower limbs is frequent and associated with pulmonary embolism. It is characterised by swelling, discolouration, superficial venous dilatation and increased temperature of the affected limb (Fig. 68). Venous thrombosis is common within the hospital population and diagnosis on clinical grounds is notoriously inaccurate. Thermography, fibrinogen scanning and venography are all techniques useful in the diagnosis of deep venous thrombosis. Thrombophlebitis (Fig. 69) is also common and usually idiopathic, but may complicate malignancy, (such as pancreatic carcinoma), sites of indwelling intravenous canulae or intravenous drug abuse.

Lymphatics

Lymphangitis may be associated with focal infection and the distribution of inflammation outlines the lymphatic vessels to the regional lymph nodes. Lymphatic obstruction, such as that associated with radical mastectomy, gives rise to distal swelling of the limb. In Milroy's disease, congenital abnormality in the lymphatics of the lower limb (Fig. 70) gives rise to chronic, non-pitting oedema of one or both legs.

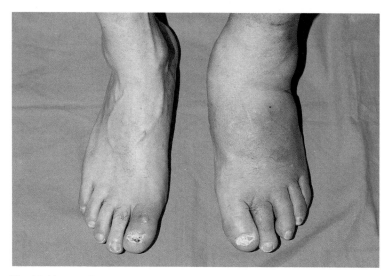

Fig. 68 Venous thrombosis.

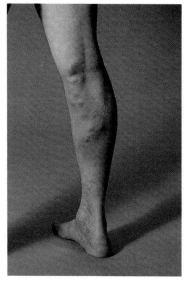

Fig. 69 Thrombophlebitis.

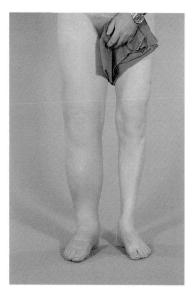

Fig. 70 Milroy's disease.

3 | Respiratory Disease (1)

Chronic obstructive lung disease

Prevalence

Chronic bronchitis and emphysema are the commonest chest disorders in Western Society, correlating largely with smoking.

Pathogenesis

Cigarette smoke causes bronchoconstriction by increased mucus production and hypertrophy of mucus glands and bronchial smooth muscle. Smoking also potentiates proteolysis within the lung, contributing to emphysema.

Clinical features

Initially, a productive morning cough and later exertional dyspnoea and infections. Central cyanosis and chest hyperinflation (Fig. 71), including intercostal indrawing, reduced chest expansion, loss of cardiac dullness, reduced crico-sternal distance and increased xiphisternal angle are also apparent. Patients with the 'blue and bloating' variety have signs of RV hypertrophy and failure. 'Pink and puffing' patients have normal Pao_2 levels with the pathological changes of emphysema. Copious sputum production is a feature of bronchiectasis (Fig. 72).

Investigations

Clinical history; chest X-ray; sputum culture; respiratory function tests, such as the FEV1/FVC ratio and the peak flow rate (PFR); and arterial blood gas analysis.

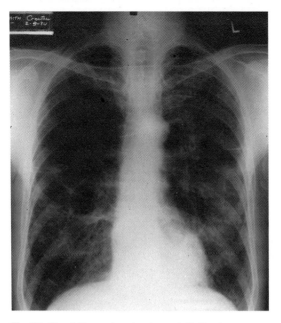

Fig. 71 Chest X-ray showing hyperinflation in emphysema.

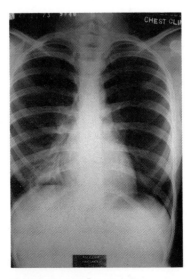

Fig. 72 Chest X-ray showing bronchiectasis.

Asthma

Prevalence

Asthma is common, affecting approximately 4% of children and 1% of adults.

Aetiology

Two types are recognised:
1. *Atopic:* due to an allergic precipitant (most often the house dust mite). The condition usually starts in childhood and is associated with eczema.
2. *Non-atopic:* in which a causal allergen cannot be found.

Clinical features

Symptoms: dyspnoea and wheeze are the cardinal symptoms. The wheeze is often worst in the morning and may be precipitated by exercise, and, occasionally, a silent chest may be apparent.

tachycardia, pulsus paradoxus, difficulty speaking and, occasionally, a silent chest may be apparent. The accessory muscles of respiration are frequently fixed to aid breathing (Fig. 73).

Investigations

PFR and FEV1, response to bronchodilators, CXR, skin tests (Fig. 74), eosinophil count, aspergillus antibody titres and blood gas analysis (in an acute attack).

Treatment

Inhalers of bronchodilators to control symptoms and steroids to reduce the frequency of attacks are sufficient in most patients. Oral steroids are required in those with more severe disease.

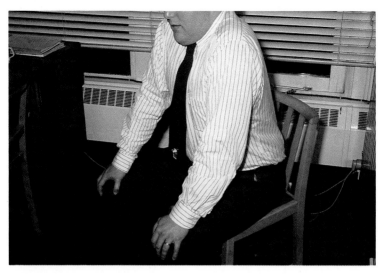

Fig. 73 Asthmatic posture with fixed accessory muscles of respiration to aid breathing.

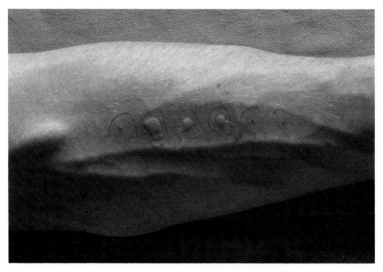

Fig. 74 Positive skin test, in an atopic subject, to a variety of common allergens.

| # Respiratory Disease (3)

Bronchogenic carcinoma

Epidemiology

Bronchogenic carcinoma is the commonest cause of death from malignancy in the UK, with an annual incidence of approximately 50 cases 100 000. Cigarette smoking is the most important risk factor, although occupational exposure to asbestos and nickel are important in some cases.

Clinical features

Symptoms: may be due to local invasion, metastatic disease or para-neoplastic syndromes. Although haemoptysis is the most important symptom, often associated with cough or chest pain, it is frequently asymptomatic in the early stages. Other symptoms include stridor, hoarseness and weight loss.
Signs: finger clubbing, cervical lymphadenopathy, signs of pulmonary collapse and/or consolidation, SVC obstruction (Fig. 75), Horner's syndrome and hepatomegaly.

Investigations

PA chest X-ray (Figs. 76 & 77) with lateral, sputum cytology, fibreoptic bronchoscopy, CT scanning of head and thorax (where indicated) and isotopic bone and liver scan.

Treatment

Surgical resection, radiotherapy and chemotherapy all have a place, depending upon the type and size of the tumour. The prognosis for the majority of patients is however, poor.

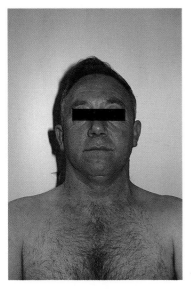

Fig. 75 Superior venacaval obstruction.

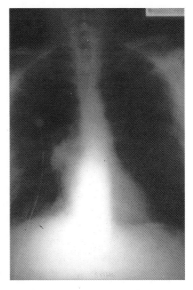

Fig. 76 Bronchogenic carcinoma at right hilum.

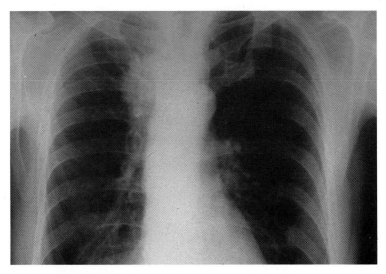

Fig. 77 Bronchogenic carcinoma in right upper lobe.

3 | Respiratory Disease (4)

Pneumonia

Pneumonia is a common disease, but the type and severity varies widely with the organism involved and the patient's age and health.

Aetiology

Common organisms involved include:
1. *Streptococcus pneumonia*.
2. *Haemophilus influenzae*.
3. Mycoplasma.
4. *Staphylococcus aureus*.
5. Legionella.

Clinical features

Symptoms: cough productive of purulent sputum, dyspnoea, pleuritic chest pain, sweats and rigors. Bronchopneumonia in the elderly may be accompanied by few symptoms other than drowsiness and confusion.
Signs: oral herpes simplex (Fig. 78), fever, reduced chest expansion, dull percussion note, coarse crepitations, bronchial breath sounds and a pleuritic rub.
   Unusual organisms producing atypical symptoms may be found in patients who are immunosuppressed.

Investigations

Sputum microscopy and culture, chest X-ray (Figs. 79 & 80), blood cultures and Mantoux test (in selected cases).

Treatment

Antibiotics effective against the organism responsible, chest physiotherapy and oxygen where required.

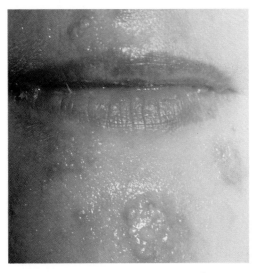

Fig. 78 Oral herpes simplex in pneumonia.

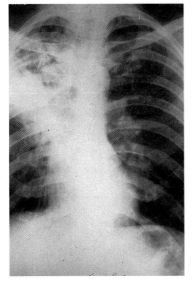

Fig. 79 Pneumonia shown in right upper zone on PA chest X-ray.

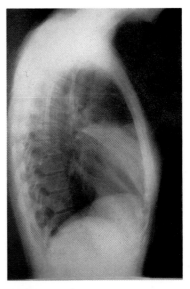

Fig. 80 Pneumonia of right middle lobe on a lateral chest X-ray.

Diffuse pulmonary fibrosis

Definition and Classification

Diffuse pulmonary fibrosis is the result of an increase in the perivascular and alveolar interstitial space, and can arise in such conditions as pneumoconiosis, sarcoidosis (Fig. 81), connective tissue disease, drug toxicity, radiation pneumonitis, tuberculosis and organic dust exposure. Many of these disorders can produce similar symptoms, signs and radiological changes, and the importance of a thorough clinical history cannot be over emphasised. Where no cause is identified, the term cryptogenic fibrosing alveolitis is used.

Fibrosing alveolitis
The majority have finger clubbing at presentation, and auscultation reveals fine crepitations. Cyanosis and cor pulmonale develop as the disease progresses. The chest X-ray may initially be normal, but later a diffuse bilateral reticulonodular pattern emerges (Figs. 82 & 83).

Extrinsic allergic alveolitis
This is due to the inhalation of organic dusts which produce a type III allergic reaction. Acute exposure produces breathlessness and cough, whilst chronic exposure may cause pulmonary fibrosis. Examples include *farmer's* and *bird-fancier's lung* and bagassosis.

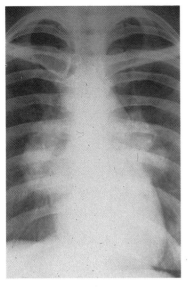

Fig. 81 Chest X-ray showing bilateral hilar lymphadenopathy in sarcoidosis.

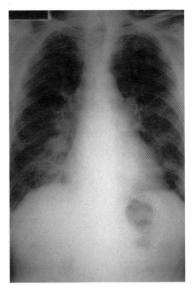

Fig. 82 Chest X-ray in Fibrosing alveolitis showing bilateral reticulonodular shadowing.

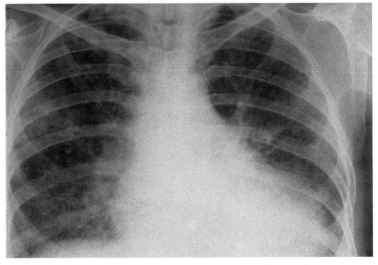

Fig. 83 Chest X-ray in fibrosing alveolitis accompanied by cardiomegaly.

Tuberculosis

Pulmonary tuberculosis remains a major health problem in developing countries. In the UK, it is still seen amongst immigrants, the elderly and in immunosuppressed subjects, including AIDS patients.

Primary tuberculous infection is usually asymptomatic, but may be associated with erythema nodosum, pleural effusion and miliary TB. Postprimary TB is the commonest type seen in the UK. It also may be asymptomatic or present with weight loss, tiredness, night sweats and haemoptysis. Apical scarring on chest X-ray should be looked for specifically (Fig. 84) and may only be apparent on special apical views.

Sarcoidosis

Sarcoidosis is a relatively common systemic granulomatous disorder of unknown cause.

Breathlessness, fever and weight loss are common presenting symptoms. Bilateral hilar lymphadenopathy is characteristic, as is erythema nodosum (Fig. 85) and polyarthralgia. A maculopapular rash, pulmonary nodules, lupus pernio and uveitis may be present. The Kveim test (Fig. 86) may be useful in difficult cases.

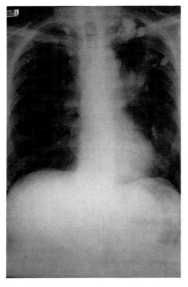

Fig. 84 Apical scarring on chest X-ray as seen in tuberculosis.

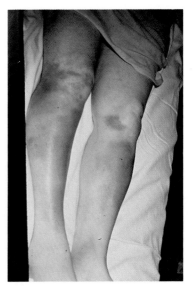

Fig. 85 Erythema nodosum characteristic of tuberculosis.

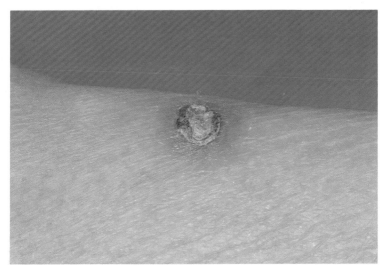

Fig. 86 Markedly positive Kveim test.

Gastrointestinal and Renal Disorders (1)

Liver

Liver disease is common with approximately 15/100 000 new cases of cirrhosis per year. In the UK, about half of these will be alcoholic, and many more patients exist with liver disease without cirrhosis. It is important to recognise these patients, as treatment (including hepatic transplantation) exists for many disorders. In all patients with liver disease, the alcohol consumption should always be asked and confirmed by relatives if alcohol abuse is suspected.

Symptoms: include RUQ discomfort, pruritus (due to cholestasis), lethargy, bruising, ankle or abdominal swelling, haematemesis, jaundice and drowsiness. Many patients with liver disease are asymptomatic and present with complications of cirrhosis such as variceal haemorrhage.
Signs: include hepatosplenomegaly, gynaecomastia (Fig. 87), spider naevi (Fig. 88) believed to be due to abnormal oestrogen metabolism, palmar erythema, testicular atrophy, loss of body hair, scratch marks (Fig. 89), parotid swelling, peripheral oedema, finger clubbing and leukonychia (Fig. 90).

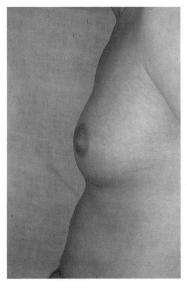

Fig. 87 Gynaecomastia seen in liver disease.

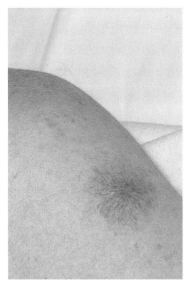

Fig. 88 A large spider naevus in a patient with cirrhosis.

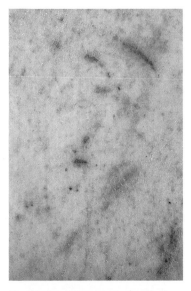

Fig. 89 Scratch marks in a patient with cholestatic liver disease.

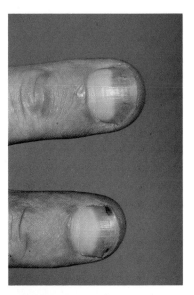

Fig. 90 Leukonychia, characteristic of cirrhosis.

Gastrointestinal and Renal Disorders (2)

Liver (contd)

Other features of liver disease which indicate liver failure include easy bruising (Fig. 91), coagulopathy and ascites (Fig. 92). Ascites may, or may not, be associated with peripheral oedema. Other signs of hepatic decompensation include jaundice and encephalopathy. Decompensation of liver function may be due to end-stage liver disease, acute or chronic liver disease, precipitated by such factors as a variceal haemorrhage, or acute liver failure. Certain features of liver disease are relatively specific to the underlying cause, such as xanthelasma associated with chronic cholestasis (Fig. 93). Splenomegaly in liver disease is rarely gross and is due to portal hypertension.

Investigations

1. Full blood count (FBC), Liver function test (LFT) and coagulation, autoantibody and virology screen.
2. Isotope liver scan and ultrasound.
3. Liver biopsy.
4. Upper GI endoscopy or barium swallow, to identify varices.
5. CAT scanning and angiography may be necessary to identify hepatic tumours, and in patients being considered for liver surgery.

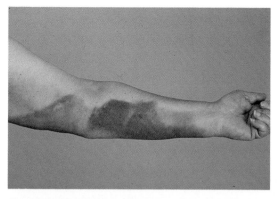

Fig. 91 Easy bruising may be a sign of liver failure.

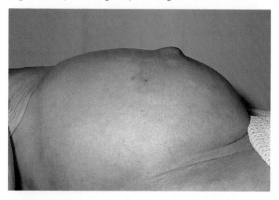

Fig. 92 Ascites.

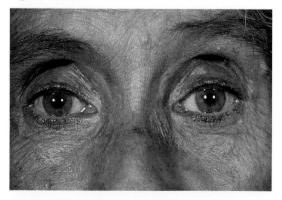

Fig. 93 Xanthelasma with chronic cholestasis.

Gastrointestinal and Renal Disorders (3)

Spleen

The normal spleen is impalpable, and it is only once it has enlarged 2–3 times normal that it can be detected by clinical examination. The spleen should be sought specifically during examination of the abdomen by bimanual palpation (Fig. 94). It can be differentiated from an enlarged left kidney by its notch, dullness to percussion, an inability to palpate above it, free movement with respiration and the presence of a space between its posterior edge and the erector spinae muscles. Where the spleen is impalpable, ultrasonic scanning can be used to accurately determine its size.

Clinical signs and associated disorders

The most frequent causes of an enlarged spleen in the UK are portal hypertension, myeloproliferative disease and myelofibrosis.

Kidneys

Examination

The kidneys are not usually palpable in healthy subjects, although in thin individuals the right kidney may be felt. They should also be specifically examined bimanually and divided into bilateral or unilateral enlargement.

1. *Bilateral enlargement:* occurs in polycystic disease, bilateral hydronephrosis and amyloidosis.
2. *Unilateral enlargement:* may be due to tumour, unilateral hydronephrosis or vicarial enlargement of the uninvolved kidney in renal artery stenosis.

Evidence of recent peritoneal dialysis or CAPD cannulae (Fig. 95) may be obvious, and haematuria should always be screened for (Fig. 96).

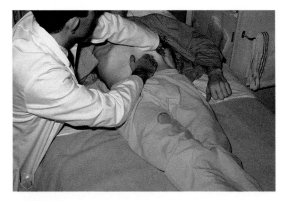

Fig. 94 Palpating for the spleen.

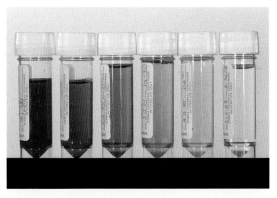

Fig. 95 Tenchkoff catheter in situ for CAPD.

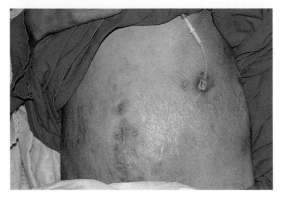

Fig. 96 Serial samples of urine showing decreasing severities of haematuria, from left to right.

4 | Gastrointestinal and Renal Disorders (4)

Scars

The abdomen should be closely inspected for scars, and, if found, their site, age and condition determined. The position of many scars provides information as to the type of surgery, such as the vertical epigastric scar of gastric surgery and the RUQ scar of cholecystectomy. The presence of numerous scars should suggest such conditions as Crohn's disease, Munchausen's syndrome or porphyria. The age of a scar can usually be determined approximately, especially if relatively recent. The presence of keloid, non-resorbable suture, drain-hole scars and the puckering of wound infection should be recorded. Occasionally, pigmentation occurs and should suggest adrenal insufficiency.

Herniae

These should be sought around scars (Fig. 97) in the inguinal and femoral region, around the umbilicus and midline (Fig. 98). They may not be visible when the patient is supine and should be palpated with the patients standing and coughing. If they contain bowel, reducability and tenderness should be tested for. If obstruction occurs, such signs as vomiting, hyperactive bowel sounds and fluid levels on an erect abdominal film may be present.

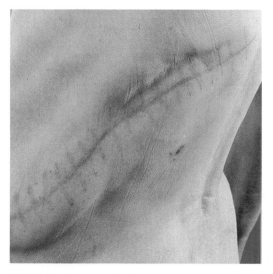

Fig. 97 Hernia secondary to surgery.

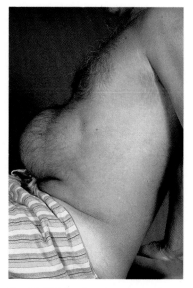

Fig. 98 Midline hernia.

Pancreas

The three main diseases of the exocrine pancreas are acute and chronic pancreatitis and pancreatic carcinoma, all of which are common and serious.

Pancreatitis

Acute pancreatitis

This is characterised by severe central abdominal pain—relieved somewhat by the patient sitting forward—and an elevated serum amylase. In the majority of cases, the causes relate to alcohol abuse or gall stones (Fig. 99). Severe attacks, which may be complicated by hypoxaemia, hypocalcaemia, disseminated intravascular coagulation and shock, have a significant mortality. Clinical signs are few, but abdominal wall bruising may appear centrally (Cullen's sign) or laterally (Grey Turner's sign) (Fig. 100) and is due to retroperitoneal haemorrhage. The formation of a pancreatic pseudocyst may follow acute pancreatitis.

Chronic pancreatitis

This may follow episodes of acute pancreatitis, or may occur without acute events. In many cases, the cause is alcohol abuse, but in others no cause can be found. The main clinical problem is chronic abdominal pain, but other complications include diabetes mellitus and steatorrhoea.

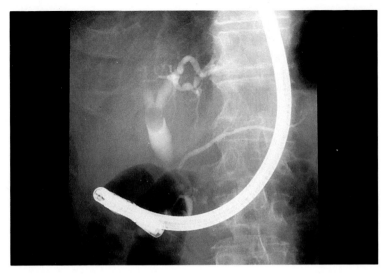

Fig. 99 An ERCP demonstrating a gallstone in the common bile duct.

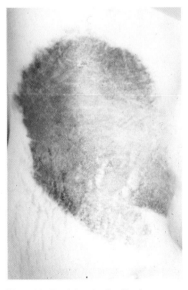

Fig. 100 Bruising in the flanks: Grey-Turner's sign.

Gastrointestinal and Renal Disorders (6)

Pancreas (contd)

Diagnosis of pancreatitis

The diagnosis is based on clinical history, pancreatic function tests and radiology, including a plain abdominal film for pancreatic calcification (Fig. 101), and ERCP.

Pancreatic cancer

Prevelance and aetiology

This is common and appears to be increasing in frequency as the population ages. The aetiology in the majority is unknown, although smoking and alcohol abuse are suspects.

Clinical features

Symptoms and signs tend to occur late in the disease with weight loss and painless obstructive jaundice. Periampullary tumours, some within the head of the gland, may present early with jaundice. The presence of a palpable gall bladder in such patients is more suggestive of carcinoma than gall stones (Courvoisier's law).

Diagnosis

The diagnosis is best made by CAT scanning, ERCP or precutaneous cholangiography (Fig. 102). Ultrasonic scanning may detect a mass within the gland, but even if this is not identified, useful information regarding the presence of stones and dilatation of the common bile duct may be obtained.

Treatment

Despite advances in diagnosis in the majority, curative surgery is not possible and palliation for jaundice and itch is all that can be offered. This is now commonly performed endoscopically by biliary stenting.

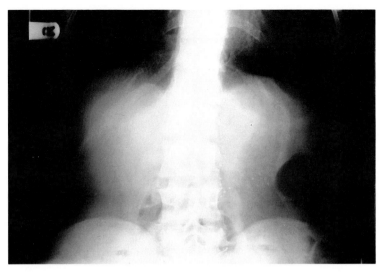

Fig. 101 Pancreatic calcification typical of alcohol-related pancreatitis.

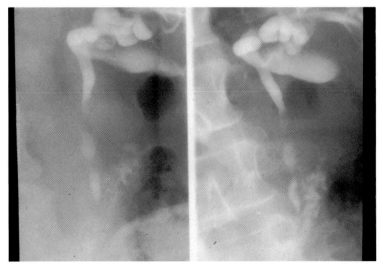

Fig. 102 A percutaneous cholangiogram showing biliary dilitation secondary to pancreatic cancer.

Inflammatory bowel disease

Incidence and aetiology

Both ulcerative colitis and Crohn's disease are common and frequently affect young people. The cause of both is unknown, although an immunological component is believed important. Crohn's disease may affect any part of the GI tract (Fig. 103), while ulcerative colitis only involves the colon.

Symptoms and signs

Although both may present with bloodly diarrhoea, abdominal pain is common only in Crohn's disease. This latter is often discovered first at laparotomy for suspected appendicitis. Apart from signs directly related to bowel disease, such as toxic dilatation in colitis, numerous systemic features may be present and include: arthritis, iritis, pyoderma gangrenosum (Fig. 104), finger clubbing and jaundice due to chronic active hepatitis or sclerosing cholangitis (Fig. 105).

Investigations

1. FBC, platelets, ESR, and LFT's.
2. Radiology and endoscopy (plus biopsies) are required for diagnosis and follow up in the majority. Close endoscopic follow up of patients with pan-colitis for longer than 12 years is essential since the risk of colonic carcinoma is increased.

Treatment

In ulcerative colitis, salazopyrin reduces the frequency of attacks. Steroids are effective in both Crohn's disease and ulcerative colitis in controlling symptoms during exacerbations.

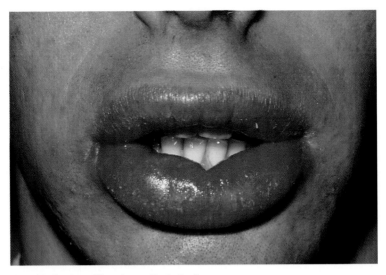

Fig. 103 Oral swelling due to Crohn's disease.

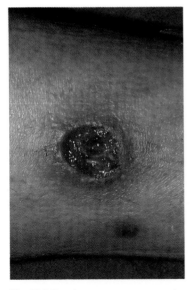

Fig. 104 Pyoderma gangrenosum in bowel disease.

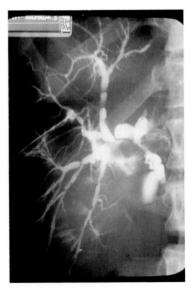

Fig. 105 A percutaneous cholangiogram in sclerosing cholangitis showing the irregularity in the biliary tree.

Gastrointestinal and Renal Disorders (8)

Gastrointestinal bleeding

Incidence

Gastrointestinal haemorrhage is common, and acute bleeding is more frequent from the upper than the lower GI tract.

Aetiology

Upper GI tract
Common causes include peptic ulceration (Fig. 106), gastric erosions, Mallory-Weis tears and oesophageal varices (Fig. 107) The history may help seperate these causes before investigation. Examination may also help clarify the likely diagnosis (e.g. hepatomegaly), but should primarily be directed towards assessing the severity of the blood loss.

Clinical features

Signs include tachycardia, hypotension, sweating, cold peripheries, pallor and confusion. Anaemia may not be present initially until haemodilution occurs.

Management

Resuscitation, surgical consultation, balloon tamponade (Fig. 108) and/or sclerotherapy of varices and, in appropriate cases, sclerotherapy of peptic ulcers. Surgery may be necessary for many patients in whom rebleeding occurs in hospital. The elderly require special care as rebleeding carries a high mortality. Treatment with ulcer-healing drugs has little influence in managing acute bleeding episodes, although maintenance therapy should reduce their frequency.

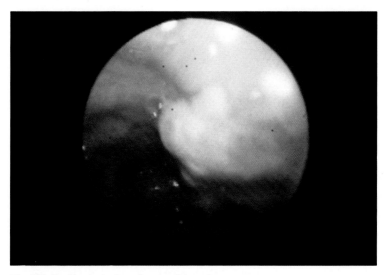

Fig. 106 Peptic ulceration shown with endoscopy.

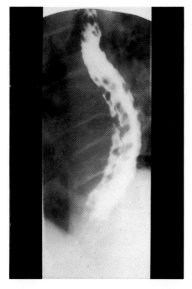

Fig. 107 A barium swallow showing filling defects in the oesophagus due to varices.

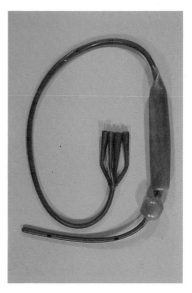

Fig. 108 A Minnesota tube.

Gastrointestinal and Renal Disorders (9)

Gastrointestinal bleeding (contd)

Lower GI tract
Bleeding from the lower GI tract usually presents with blood rectally, but not melaena.

Aetiology

Causes include haemorrhoids, diverticular disease, inflammatory bowel disease, ischaemic colitis, malignancy (Fig. 109) and vascular malformations (Fig. 110). This last is particularly common from the right side of the colon, and in the elderly.

Clinical features

Although torrential bleeding is less common in the lower GI than upper GI tract, it may be equally life threatening. Often bleeding is chronic and occult, the patient presenting with iron-deficient anaemia.

Management

1. *Resuscitation and surgical consultation:* if acute rectal bleeding.
2. *Sigmoidoscopy or colonoscopy:* to assess site of bleeding.
3. *Angiography:* may be required to identify site of bleeding from vascular malformations.
4. *Laparotomy and segmental colonic resection:* may be indicated in emergencies.
   Bleeding due to inflammatory bowel disease usually responds to bed rest and steroids.

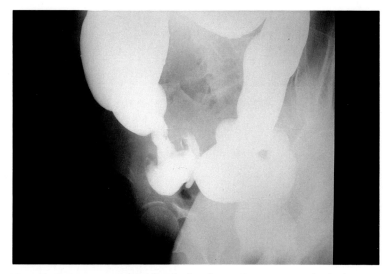

Fig. 109 Barium enema showing the 'apple-core' appearance of colonic carcinoma.

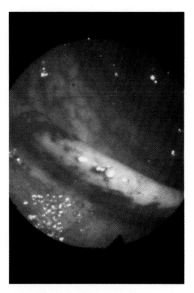

Fig. 110 The colonoscopic appearance of angiodysplasia in the colon.

4 | Gastrointestinal and Renal Disorders (10)

Acute abdominal pain

Examination

When examining a patient with abdominal pain, it is essential to identify the site of maximal pain. Examination should be careful so as not to cause excessive pain, and the patient should be asked initially to indicate the tender area. This alone will often provide clues as to the diagnosis, such as the pointing sign of peptic ulceration (Fig. 111).

When a site of pain is found, rebound tenderness—elicited by compression at a site distant from the original site followed by sudden release—should be sought. If present, such tenderness indicates peritoneal involvement. Visceral rupture with generalised peritonitis is almost always associated with a rigid abdomen and absent bowel sounds, although these signs may not be present in the elderly and in patients on steroid therapy. Other causes include pancreatitis, obstruction (Fig. 112), hypercalcaemia (Fig. 113) and ketoacidosis.

Investigations

1. Chest X-ray to identify air under the diaphragm.
2. Erect and supine abdominal film to identify intestinal obstruction and its site.
3. Haemoglobin, white cell count, LFT's, calcium, glucose and amylase.
4. Ultrasound and contrast radiology.

In some patients, further investigation fails to identify a cause of abdominal pain and the irritable bowel syndrome is presumed to be the cause.

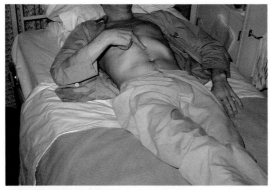

Fig. 111 Patient indicating area of pain in peptic ulceration.

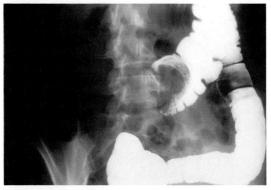

Fig. 112 A barium enema illustrating intussusception.

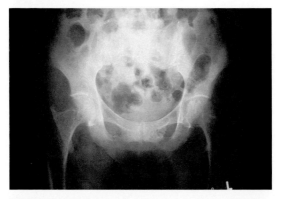

Fig. 113 Pelvic X-ray in hyperparathyroidism showing patchy bone resorbtion.

Gastrointestinal and Renal Disorders (11)

Diarrhoea

The frequent passage of soft or liquid stools is a common problem and only infrequently indicates serious disease. Chronicity and the passage of blood require investigation.

Bloody diarrhoea

Causes of bloody diarrhoea include inflammatory bowel disease, infective diarrhoea, ischaemic colitis, colonic carcinoma and pseudomembranous colitis (Fig. 114).

Steatorrhoea

This is the passage of usually bulky, offensive stool which floats. Causes include pancreatic insufficiency, enteropathy (e.g. coeliac disease), giardiasis (Fig. 115) and bacterial overgrowth which is more likely after gastric surgery and with bowel disease (Fig. 116).

Watery diarrhoea

This is often infective, but may be due to irritable bowel syndrome, constipation with overflow, laxative abuse and many other conditions (e.g. cholera, drug reaction and thyrotoxicosis).

Variable diarrhoea and constipation

In patients with the irritable bowel syndrome, alternating diarrhoea and constipation is common. The diarrhoea is seldom nocturnal and never contains blood.

Investigations

Stool culture, white blood cell count, sigmoidoscopy and biopsy, abdominal film, contrast radiology, and hydrogen breath test.

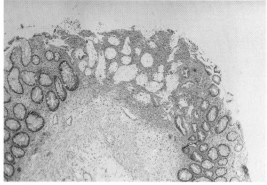

Fig. 114 A photomicrograph of pseudomembranous colitis.

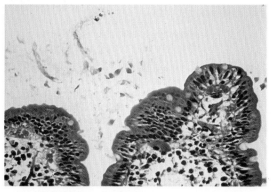

Fig. 115 A photomicrograph of jejunal giardiasis.

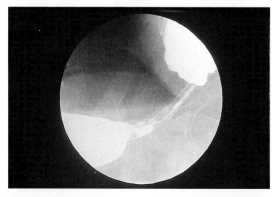

Fig. 116 A tight stricture in a patient with scleroderma.

Gastrointestinal and Renal Disorders (12)

Dysphagia

The sensation of difficulty in swallowing or of food sticking is important and requires investigation.

Clinical features

The site at which the patient feels food sticking bears little relation to the site of obstruction. The duration and type of onset (whether for all food or just solids) should be determined. A past history of reflux oesophagitis suggests a benign peptic stricture. Associated features, such as lymphadenopathy, epigastric mass and pulmonary aspiration, should be sought.

Causes

These include benign peptic strictures, oesophageal carcinoma (Fig. 117), achalasia (Fig. 118), dysmotility, severe oesophagitis (Fig. 119), pharyngeal pouch or diverticulum (Fig. 120). Associated iron-deficiency anaemia should raise the possibility of Plummer-Vinson syndrome in which an oesophageal web is the cause of dysphagia.

Investigations

1. Barium swallow (should precede endoscopy to identify high strictures and pharyngeal pouches).
2. Endoscopy and biopsy (and dilatation if appropriate)
   Endoscopic laser therapy may be useful in treating malignant dysphagia.

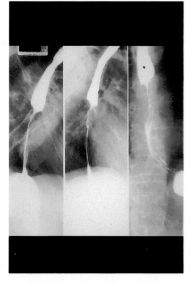

Fig. 117 Barium swallow illustrating a stricture due to oesophageal carcinoma.

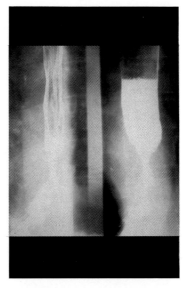

Fig. 118 Barium swallow showing typical appearance of achalasia.

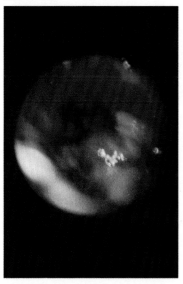

Fig. 119 Endoscopic appearance of severe oesophagitis.

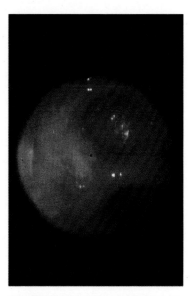

Fig. 120 Endoscopic appearance of an oesophageal diverticulum.

Gastrointestinal and Renal Disorders (13)

Vomiting

The causes of vomiting are miriad, but can be broadly divided into central, local, obstructive and systemic. Many are relatively unimportant, but vomiting may herald serious disease.

Clinical features

Where possible, the vomit should be inspected for blood, food contents and bile. The patient should be questioned about associated nausea, drugs, CNS and GI symptoms, although renal and endocrine diseases may be responsible. Pregnancy and alcohol abuse should not be forgotten as a cause. Examination should look for signs of cardiac and renal failure. The abdomen should be inspected for epigastric tenderness and masses. Obstruction may be obvious with prominant peristaltic waves. Eliciting a succussion splash (Fig. 121) is only of significance in a patient fasting for two or more hours.

Investigations

1. Treatment of dehydration with intravenous fluids and nasogastric suction where appropriate.
2. Erect and supine X-rays (Fig. 122).
3. Contrast radiology or endoscopy.
   Other tests may incude head CAT scan, electrolytes and LFT's, and serum drug level determination.

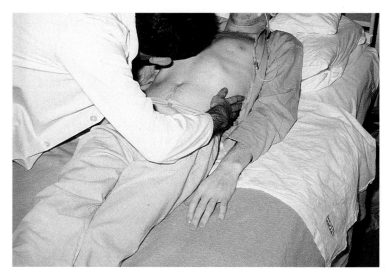

Fig. 121 Technique for eliciting a succussion splash.

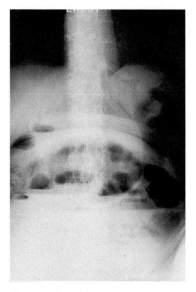

Fig. 122 Erect X-ray demonstrating numerous fluid levels.

Gastrointestinal and Renal Disorders (14)

Rectal examination

The rectal examination is an integral part of the complete medical examination. In combination with proctoscopy, it will detect internal and external haemorrhoids, prostatic hypertrophy and carcinoma, and the majority of rectal tumours. Local lesions such as anal fissures, warts and abscesses (Fig. 123) should be recorded.

Examination

The procedure should be explained to the patient before being undertaken. The subject should adopt the left lateral position, and the buttocks and anus examined. Adequate lubricating jelly should be applied before the gloved finger is slowly inserted. The tone of the anal sphincter around the finger should be assessed. Palpation should be systematic of all four quadrants, and faecal material should be tested for faecal occult blood after withdrawal. Haemorrhoids, unless thrombosed, are not palpable and are detected by proctoscopy. Rectal prolapse can only be excluded after getting the patient to bear down (Figs. 124 & 125).

The presence of haemorrhoids should not be assumed to be the cause of rectal bleeding, particularly if the blood is mixed throughout the stool.

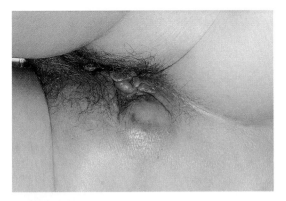

Fig. 123 Peri-anal abscess.

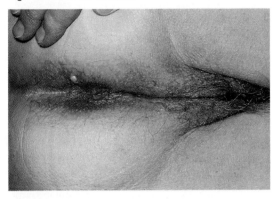

Fig. 124 Inspection of the anus at rest.

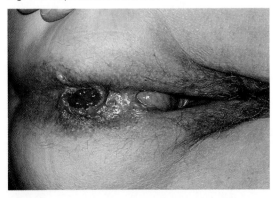

Fig. 125 Inspection of the anus during a valsalva manoeuvre.

5 | Central Nervous System Disorders (1)

Cerebrovascular disease

Prevalence

In the UK, approximately 100 000 patients suffer their first stroke each year.

Pathogenesis

Cerebral infarction due to thrombosis or embolism is the commonest cause. Cerebral haemorrhage (Fig. 126) is less common and is usually related to hypertension and/or an aneurysm (Fig. 127).

Clinical features

These relate to the affected territory of the cerebrum, cerebellum or brain stem.
1. *Middle cerebral artery* involvement is the most common, causing hemiplegia.
2. *Anterior cerebral artery* involvement causes hemiplegia with the leg weaker than the arm, with or without expressive dysphasia.
3. *Posterior cerebral artery* involvement often produces a contralateral homonymous hemianopia with macular sparing.
   A crossed paralysis with ipsilateral cranial nerve involvement (Fig. 128) suggests a brain stem lesion, whilst vertigo, ataxia, vomiting and nystagmus occur with cerebellar damage.

Risk factors

Age, hypertension, atrial fibrillation, ischaemic heart disease and diabetes mellitus.

Treatment

Unfortunately, this is poor in the majority, and prevention is where efforts should be concentrated. In patients with cerebral embolism, the source should be identified and treated if possible. Anticoagulation is advocated for patients at risk, such as those with mitral valve disease and atrial fibrillation. Neurosurgery should be considered in those with cerebral haemorrhage if the CAT scan reveals it to be accessible.

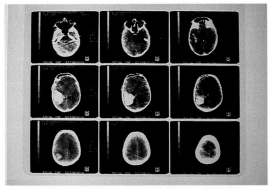

Fig. 126 The CAT appearance of a right occipito-parietal haemorrhage.

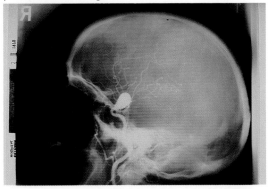

Fig. 127 An angiogram showing a large intracranial aneurysm.

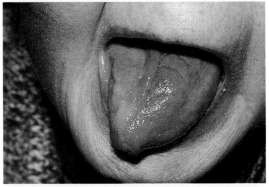

Fig. 128 Appearance of tongue in right 12th cranial nerve lesion.

Central Nervous System Disorders (2)

Multiple sclerosis

This is a disease of unknown cause which results in multiple areas of demyelination throughout the CNS. The NMR scan has sufficient definition to show small areas of demyelination and aids early diagnosis (Fig. 129).

Clinical features

The symptoms are numerous, but patients often present with blurred vision, or temporary weakness or paraesthesia in a limb.

Prognosis

These symptoms are often transient, but with time, severe neurological deficit accrues leaving the patient wheelchair-bound and leading to early death.

Neuropathies

The term neuropathy is used to describe all disorders of nerves outside of the brain and spinal cord. Classification is based on anatomical position and sensory, motor or mixed nerve involvement.

Peripheral neuropathy
Peripheral nerve fibres are affected, and the usual presentation is of a symmetrical, mixed sensory-motor neuropathy affecting the distal aspect of the limbs (Fig. 130). The commonest cause is diabetes mellitus, but the condition is also seen with carcinoma, vitamin B_{12} and B_1 deficiency, uraemia, drug toxicity and Guillan-Barre syndrome.

Mononeuropathy
Pressure or trauma is the commonest cause of abnormality of one nerve, with the radial and ulnar being the commonest examples (Fig. 131).

Mononeuritis multiplex
This is a disorder affecting at least two nerves concurrently or serially. The symptoms are paraesthesia and pain, with associated weakness or wasting. It is most often due to diabetes.

CLINICAL SIGNS

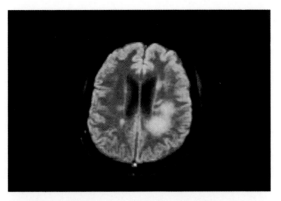

Fig. 129 An NMR scan in multiple sclerosis.

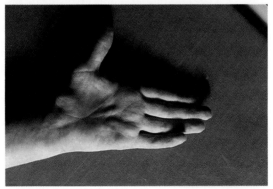

Fig. 130 Appearance of the hand in a patient with peripheral neuropathy.

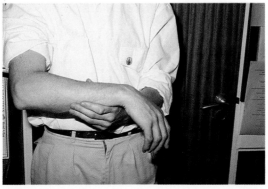

Fig. 131 Wrist drop typical of radial nerve palsy.

**General
Examination**

The musculoskeletal system should be examined
systematically, looking at static posture, walking
and bending, and individual joints. The latter
should be observed at rest, and with both passive
and active movement.

**Common
disorders**

The commonest disorders include rheumatoid
arthritis, osteoarthrosis, gout and ankylosing
spondylitis.

Rheumatoid disease
The commonest joints involved are the hands and
feet (Fig. 132). The ankles and elbows should be
inspected (with particular attention to the latter)
for rheumatoid nodules. Associated signs include
vasculitis, splenomegaly, pulmonary crepitations
with fibrosing alveolitis, carpal tunnel syndrome,
pericarditis, lymphadenopathy and
keratoconjunctivitis sicca. Examination of the
neck, particularly radiology, is important before
such procedures as endoscopy and general
anaesthesia can be performed looking for
instability of the cervical vertebrae.

Osteoarthrosis
Primary osteoarthrosis is commoner in females
and is usually visible in the hand (Fig. 133), where
Heberden's nodes are the characteristic finding.
These are osteophytes on the dorsal surface of
the terminal phalanges.

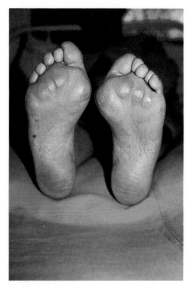

Fig. 132 Rheumatoid feet showing callous over the metatarsal heads.

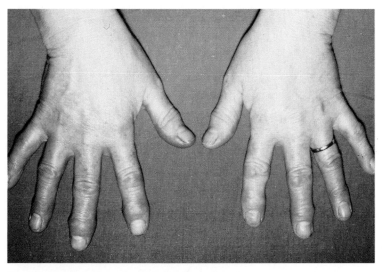

Fig. 133 Heberden's nodes seen in osteoarthrosis.

Common disorders (contd)

Secondary osteoarthrosis
This is commoner in males, most often affecting the cervical spine, lumbar spine, knees and hips. Joint involvement is usually asymmetrical. Radiology frequently identifies osteoarthrosis without symptoms, particularly in the neck.

Ankylosing spondylitis
This condition is far commoner in males and is associated strongly with HLA B27. It usually affects the sacroiliac spine early, with stiffness and low back pain, and later the thoracic and cervical spine.

Gout
This affects males more than females and is familial. It is characterised by episodes of acute arthritis, initially of single joints associated with hyperuricaemia. The great toe is involved in 75% of cases (Fig. 134), but the hands may also be involved (Fig. 135). The diagnosis is confirmed by the typical features, in conjunction with a high serum urate level.

Chondrocalcinosis
This condition, also known as pseudogout, is due to calcium pyrophosphate deposition and affects the knee most commonly (Fig. 136).

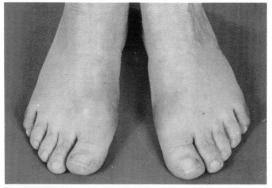

Fig. 134 Erythema over the base of the great toe in acute gout.

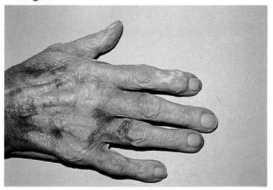

Fig. 135 Gout involving the hands.

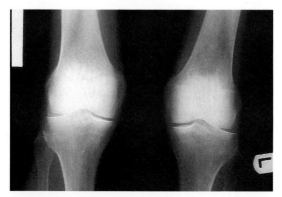

Fig. 136 Radiological appearance of chondrocalcinosis in a patient with hyperparathyroidism.

Adrenal Disease

Cushing's syndrome

Overproduction of cortisol from the adrenal cortex may occur because of adrenal disease (such as adrenal adenoma or carcinoma) or secondary to excessive ACTH from the pituitary (Cushing's disease), or from ACTH-producing tumours. In advanced Cushing's syndrome, the signs are obvious, with central obesity (Fig. 137), striae (Fig. 138), hypertension, hyperglycaemia, plethoric (moon) face, proximal myopathy and a buffalo hump. In milder cases, these signs may be absent or subtle. Measurement of diurnal serum cortisol levels (and ACTH) is required for the diagnosis.

Addison's disease

Underactivity of the adrenal cortex may occur because of rapid withdrawal of steroid therapy or, less often, because of adrenal damage (Addison's disease). The former may present as a medical emergency with collapse. Addison's disease is most often due to autoimmune distruction, but also occurs as a result of metastatic disease and tuberculosis. It presents insidiously with signs of lethargy, hypotension, weight loss and pigmentation. This latter occurs in the skin creases, scars, light-exposed areas and the oral mucus membranes (Fig. 139). Although hyperkalaemia is typical of hypoadrenalism, a synacthen test is required for the diagnosis.

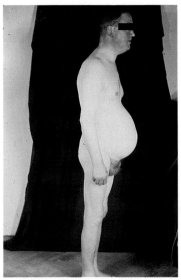

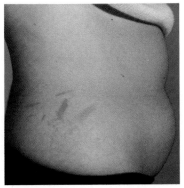

Fig. 137 Lateral view of patient with Cushing's syndrome, showing central obesity and thin limbs with proximal myopathy.

Fig. 138 Striae seen in Cushing's syndrome.

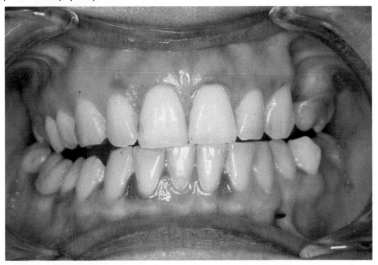

Fig. 139 Patches of pigmentation of the oral mucus membranes seen in Addison's disease.

Diabetes mellitus

Diabetes mellitus is a common disease in Western Society which may be either primary, and of unknown cause, or secondary to such underlying disorders as chronic pancreatitis, Cushing's syndrome and acromegaly. The long-term complications cause serious morbidity and mortality.

Complications

Atheroma
This develops prematurely resulting in ischaemic heart disease, strokes and gangrene (p. 43).

Microvascular disease
This results in retinopathy (Fig. 140), currently one of the commonest causes of blindness, and renal failure in which a relatively early feature is proteinuria. It is believed that good control of the diabetes reduces the risk of developing such microvascular changes, but strong evidence for this is still lacking. Control of hypertension is an important part of the management in preventing diabetic renal disease.

Neuropathy
This commonly affects peripheral sensory nerves and presents with pain and paraesthesia. Foot ulcers are a common complication. Paraesthesia may give rise to Charcot's joints (Figs. 141 & 142) where lack of pain sensation allows continued injury to damaged tissues.

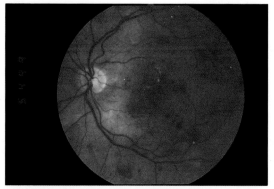

Fig. 140 Retinopathy seen in diabetes mellitus illustrating blot and dot haemorrahges.

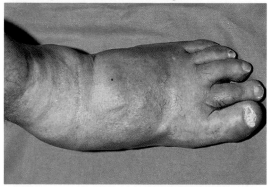

Fig. 141 Appearance of disrupted ankle joint in diabetes mellitus.

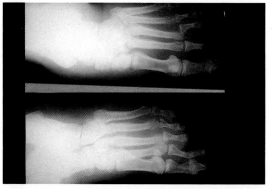

Fig. 142 Radiologic appearance of disrupted ankle joint in diabetes mellitus.

Diabetes mellitus (contd)

Complications
(contd)

Neuropathy (contd)
Neuropathy may also be present with pain and can be difficult to treat. Autonomic neuropathy may result in gastrointestinal disorders, such as diarrhoea, postural hypotension and impotence.

Skin
The cutaneous manifestations associated with diabetes mellitus may be specific, or non-specific but increased in frequency. Necrobiosis lipoidica, characterised by skin lesions of yellow-brown atrophy with sharply defined edges, occurs usually (bot not exclusively) in diabetics (Fig. 143). Boils and abscesses occur more frequently in diabetes, particularly if poorly controlled. Less common problems such as granuloma annulare occur more often in diabetic subjects (Fig. 144). Skin lesions may also develop at the site of insulin injection, either as fat hypertrophy or, more rarely nowadays, fat atrophy. Injection into such areas leads to variable insulin absorption and should be avoided.

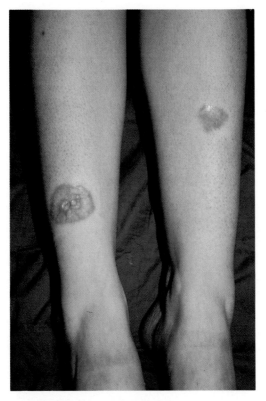

Fig. 143 Necrobiosis lipoidica in a diabetic patient.

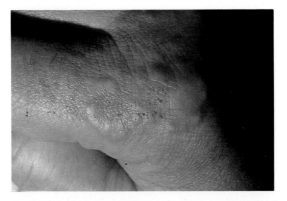

Fig. 144 Granuloma annulare: more frequent in diabetics.

Thyroid disease

Thyroid disease is particularly common in women. Although many patients demonstrate classical signs and symptoms, these may be absent in others.

Thyrotoxicosis

The commonest cause is Grave's disease, but a multinodular goitre or acute thyroiditis may occasionally be responsible.
Symptoms: include heat intolerance, weight loss, anxiety, palpitations and diarrhoea.
Signs: include goitre (Fig. 145), large pulse volume, onycholysis, lid retraction, exophthalmus and excessive sweating.

Hypothyroidism

The commonest cause is Hashimoto's autoimmune thyroiditis. It may also develop after partial thyroidectomy or drug treatment for thyrotoxicosis, or may be due to hypothalamic or pituitary disease.
Symptoms: include lethargy, constipation, cold intolerance and menorrhagia.
Signs: include hair dryness and loss, weight gain, prolonged tendon reflexes and periorbital puffiness (Fig. 146).

Investigations

Serum T3 and thyroid stimulating hormone (TSH) levels are usually sufficient. In cases where the diagnosis is not clear, radio-iodine uptake and ultrasound scans may be invaluable. In a small minority, therapeutic trials with thyroxine or antithyroid drugs, such as carbimazole, may be useful.

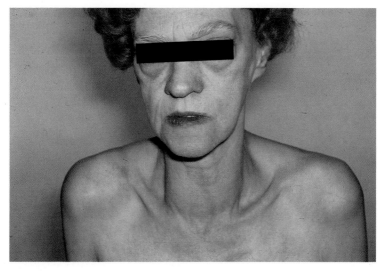

Fig. 145 Goitre seen in patient with thyrotoxicosis.

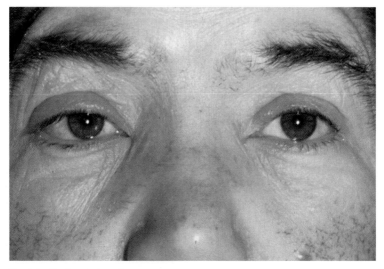

Fig. 146 Periorbital puffiness in hypothyroidism.

8 | Acquired Immunodeficiency Syndrome (1)

Aetiology and pathogenesis

AIDS is the end stage of chronic infection with the human immunodeficiency virus (HIV). Acute infection may be associated with a febrile illness, but is often asymptomatic. As the disease progresses, common infections become more frequent. Some patients develop persistent generalised lymphadenopathy. End-stage disease or AIDS is associated with certain indicator disorders which include specific opportunistic infections, unusual tumours and reduced numbers of T helper cells. In many, the diagnosis is reached by a suggestive history, such as intravenous drug abuse or homosexuality, in association with chronic ill-health.

Clinical features

Respiratory involvement
A respiratory illness is the most common presentation, with pneumocystis carinii pneumonia (PCP) being the presenting feature in 50% of all cases (Fig. 147). Atypical bacterial and viral pneumonias are also common. Pulmonary involvement with metastatic Kaposi's sarcoma is also recognised.

Gastrointestinal disease
Infection and malignancy may affect any part of the GI tract. Candida is the commonest infection of the mouth (Fig. 148), larynx and oesophagus (Fig. 149). Herpes simplex (HSV) can cause painful, recurrent oral ulceration, and Epstein-Barr virus has been implicated in oral hairy leukoplakia (Fig. 150).

CLINICAL SIGNS

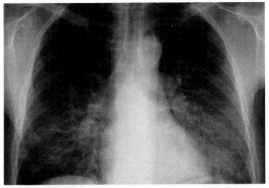

Fig. 147 Chest X-ray of pneumocystis pneumonia with the typical perihilar infiltrate.

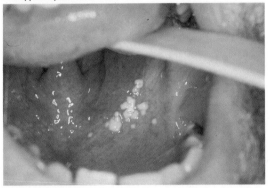

Fig. 148 Oral candida can present in AIDS.

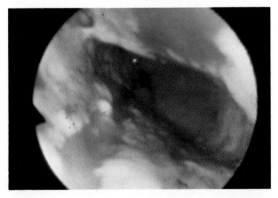

Fig. 149 Endoscopic view of oesophageal candidiasis.

Clinical features (contd)

Gastrointestinal disease (contd)
The palate may be an early site of involvement in Kaposi's sarcoma (Fig. 151). Cryptosporidium is the commonest pathogen of the small bowel, causing diarhoea, malabsorption and weight loss. The large bowel may be infected with CMV or HSV which may give rise to perianal ulceration, diagnostic of AIDS. The most common GI symptoms are: oral discomfort, dysphagia, weight loss and diarrhoea.

Skin manifestations
The skin conditions associated with AIDS are Kaposi's sarcoma (which leads to diagnosis in 25%), mucocutaneous HSV, atypical mycobacterium infection and non-Hodgkin's lymphoma. Kaposi's sarcoma initially resembles a bruise, but eventually develops into firm, purple nodules, frequently at different sites (Fig. 152).

Neurology
Encephalopathy, myelopathy and peripheral neuropathy occur, as does meningitis (*Cryptococcus neoformans*) and space-occupying lesions (Toxoplasma gondii). CMV retinitis may cause visual field loss.

Treatment

The epidemic of HIV infection is likely to increase, with patients being seen with increasing frequency in all the disciplines of medicine. Although considerable research is currently being concentrated in the treatment of AIDS, prevention remains the only 'cure'.

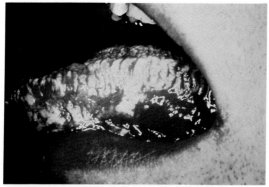

Fig. 150 Oral hairy leukoplakia may be a feature of Epstein-Barr virus infection in AIDS.

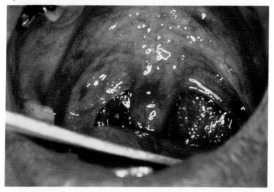

Fig. 151 Kaposi's sarcoma of the soft palate.

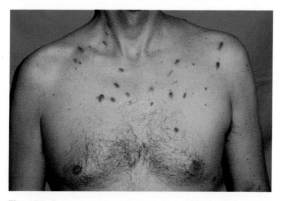

Fig. 152 Cutaneous purple nodules of Kaposi's sarcoma.

Index